Herbal Antibiotics

Learn How To Use 35 Most Common Herbal Antivirals For Safe Healing And Not To Cause Harm

Table of content

Introduction

You feel that little tickle in the back of your throat, and you sigh. You don't have time to get sick right now, and you certainly don't have time to feel groggy from your cold medicine. You have a life to live, and many things to do during your day – when are you going to have the time to sit back and be sick?

You have kids, and you know with kids that cuts and scrapes happen, and you hate risking the infection. On the other hand, you don't want to spread chemicals on your child's body when you know that it could cause other side effects – so you feel tied.

What do you do?

If only there was a way you could go all natural with your remedies. If only there was a way you could know without a doubt you were taking care of what needed to be taken care of, but you weren't bringing in harmful side effects while you did it.

If only there was a natural remedy for all the different things you and your children have to deal with during the day.

Or is there?

When you know how to use herbs for your health, you unlock the door to a whole new world. You give yourself the gift of health and healing, and you spare yourself the pain of having to deal with side effects. By taking control of your health through natural remedies, you give yourself the gift of goodness – without anything bad to go along with it.

Have you wanted to get healthy the natural way?

Have you wanted to care for scrapes and bruises without any artificial medication?

You have come to the right place. Let me show you exactly what you need to do to use herbal remedies for a variety of illnesses, and give you perfect control of your life back.

You deserve to be happy and healthy, and with these remedies, you are going to get that very thing.

Let's get started.

Chapter 1 – Herbal Healing

Herbs have been used for thousands of years because of their incredible medicinal properties. Whether you use them as a tea, or you mix them into a salve and apply to the injury itself, you are going to find all kinds of wonderful healing – from the inside out.

Mix up all these different remedies, and enjoy a kind of healing like you never imagined you could have from the natural world. Save on prescriptions. Save time not standing in line at the pharmacy, and save your health with herbs that are meant to heal!

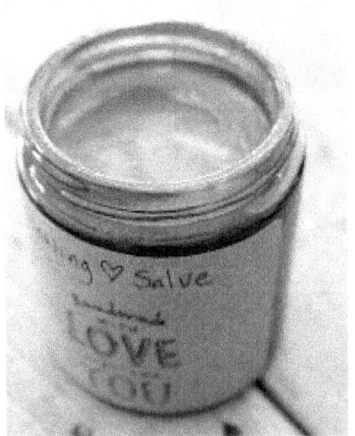

Scratch Sealer
What you will need:

3 tablespoons colloidal silver

8 drops tea tree oil

1/3 cup chopped beeswax

½ cup mango butter

Directions:

Heat 1 cup of water in a stainless steel pan on your stove. Crush the herbs and place them in the boiling water and turn the heat down to a simmer. Allow to simmer for 8 hours.

Strain the herbs out of the water and discard the herbs.

In a double boiler, melt the mango butter and beeswax. Once melted, stir in ½ cup of the herbal infused water. Add the tea tree oil next.

Once all is combined, transfer to another jar to cool.

Apply directly to infected area, and cover with a bandage. Wash the infected area with gentle soap and water and replace with more salve and a clean bandage twice per day.

Infection Fighter
What you will need:

2 tablespoons peppermint leaves

1 tablespoon grated, dried lemon peel

Directions:

Make sure all the herbs you are using are dried and clean. Crush them into smaller pieces and set aside.

Line a tea ball with a paper towel so the finer bits of the herbs do not seep out of the ball as the tea is being prepared. Mix the herbs with 1 tablespoon black tea, and transfer to the ball.

Steep in a mug of hot water for up to 10 minutes, and stir in 1 tablespoon of honey, if desired. Enjoy.

Repeat up to 3 times per day for as long as symptoms persist.

Home Doctor
What you will need:

1 tablespoon chamomile leaves

1 tablespoon licorice leaves

Directions:

Make sure all the herbs you are using are dried and clean. Crush them into smaller pieces and set aside.

Line a tea ball with a paper towel so the finer bits of the herbs do not seep out of the ball as the tea is being prepared. Mix the herbs with 1 tablespoon black tea, and transfer to the ball.

Steep in a mug of hot water for up to 10 minutes, and stir in 1 tablespoon of honey, if desired. Enjoy.

Repeat up to 3 times per day for as long as symptoms persist.

Throat Coat

What you will need:

2 cinnamon sticks, crushed

1 tablespoon lemon zest

1 tablespoon peppermint leaves

Directions:

Make sure all the herbs you are using are dried and clean. Crush them into smaller pieces and set aside.

Line a tea ball with a paper towel so the finer bits of the herbs do not seep out of the ball as the tea is being prepared. Mix the herbs with 1 tablespoon black tea, and transfer to the ball.

Steep in a mug of hot water for up to 10 minutes, and stir in 1 tablespoon of honey, if desired. Enjoy.

Repeat up to 3 times per day for as long as symptoms persist.

Universal Healer

What you will need:

2 tablespoons crushed sage leaves

1 tablespoon slippery elm

Directions:

Make sure all the herbs you are using are dried and clean. Crush them into smaller pieces and set aside.

Line a tea ball with a paper towel so the finer bits of the herbs do not seep out of the ball as the tea is being prepared. Mix the herbs with 1 tablespoon black tea, and transfer to the ball.

Steep in a mug of hot water for up to 10 minutes, and stir in 1 tablespoon of honey, if desired. Enjoy.

Repeat up to 3 times per day for as long as symptoms persist.

Joint Lube

What you will need:

3 tablespoons peppermint leaves

2 tablespoons spearmint leaves

8 drops tea tree oil

1/3 cup chopped beeswax

½ cup mango butter

Directions:

Heat 1 cup of water in a stainless steel pan on your stove. Crush the herbs and place them in the boiling water and turn the heat down to a simmer. Allow to simmer for 8 hours.

Strain the herbs out of the water and discard the herbs.

In a double boiler, melt the mango butter and beeswax. Once melted, stir in ½ cup of the herbal infused water. Add the tea tree oil next.

Once all is combined, transfer to another jar to cool.

Apply directly to infected area, and cover with a bandage. Wash the infected area with gentle soap and water and replace with more salve and a clean bandage twice per day.

Cold and Flu Buster
What you will need:

1 garlic clove

2 tablespoons red root, crushed

Directions:

Make sure all the herbs you are using are dried and clean. Crush them into smaller pieces and set aside.

Line a tea ball with a paper towel so the finer bits of the herbs do not seep out of the ball as the tea is being prepared. Mix the herbs with 1 tablespoon black tea, and transfer to the ball.

Steep in a mug of hot water for up to 10 minutes, and stir in 1 tablespoon of honey, if desired. Enjoy.

Repeat up to 3 times per day for as long as symptoms persist.

Cough Catcher
What you will need:

2 cinnamon sticks, crushed

1 tablespoon crushed dried ginger

1 tablespoon orange zest

Directions:

Make sure all the herbs you are using are dried and clean. Crush them into smaller pieces and set aside.

Line a tea ball with a paper towel so the finer bits of the herbs do not seep out of the ball as the tea is being prepared. Mix the herbs with 1 tablespoon black tea, and transfer to the ball.

Steep in a mug of hot water for up to 10 minutes, and stir in 1 tablespoon of honey, if desired. Enjoy.

Repeat up to 3 times per day for as long as symptoms persist.

All Gain No Pain

What you will need:

1 tablespoon turmeric

2 tablespoons valerian root

8 drops tea tree oil

1/3 cup chopped beeswax

½ cup mango butter

Directions:

Heat 1 cup of water in a stainless steel pan on your stove. Crush the herbs and place them in the boiling water and turn the heat down to a simmer. Allow to simmer for 8 hours.

Strain the herbs out of the water and discard the herbs.

In a double boiler, melt the mango butter and beeswax. Once melted, stir in ½ cup of the herbal infused water. Add the tea tree oil next.

Once all is combined, transfer to another jar to cool.

Apply directly to infected area, and cover with a bandage. Wash the infected area with gentle soap and water and replace with more salve and a clean bandage twice per day.

Against the Grain

What you will need:

3 tablespoons eucommia

8 drops tea tree oil

1/3 cup chopped beeswax

½ cup mango butter

Directions:

Heat 1 cup of water in a stainless steel pan on your stove. Crush the herbs and place them in the boiling water and turn the heat down to a simmer. Allow to simmer for 8 hours.

Strain the herbs out of the water and discard the herbs.

In a double boiler, melt the mango butter and beeswax. Once melted, stir in ½ cup of the herbal infused water. Add the tea tree oil next.

Once all is combined, transfer to another jar to cool.

Apply directly to infected area, and cover with a bandage. Wash the infected area with gentle soap and water and replace with more salve and a clean bandage twice per day.

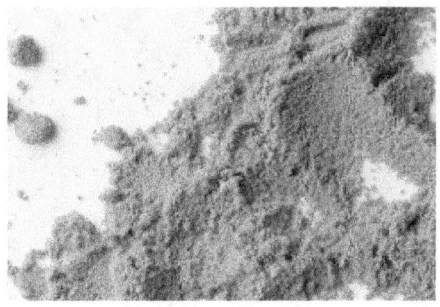

Happy Health
What you will need:

1 tablespoon clean, crushed rose hips

1 tablespoon crushed dried ginger root

Directions:

Make sure all the herbs you are using are dried and clean. Crush them into smaller pieces and set aside.

Line a tea ball with a paper towel so the finer bits of the herbs do not seep out of the ball as the tea is being prepared. Mix the herbs with 1 tablespoon black tea, and transfer to the ball.

Steep in a mug of hot water for up to 10 minutes, and stir in 1 tablespoon of honey, if desired. Enjoy.

Repeat up to 3 times per day for as long as symptoms persist.

Purity

What you will need:

2 tablespoons crushed anise seeds

1 tablespoon crushed peppermint leaves

Directions:

Make sure all the herbs you are using are dried and clean. Crush them into smaller pieces and set aside.

Line a tea ball with a paper towel so the finer bits of the herbs do not seep out of the ball as the tea is being prepared. Mix the herbs with 1 tablespoon black tea, and transfer to the ball.

Steep in a mug of hot water for up to 10 minutes, and stir in 1 tablespoon of honey, if desired. Enjoy.

Repeat up to 3 times per day for as long as symptoms persist.

Breathe Easy

What you will need:

1 teaspoon crushed dried red pepper flakes

3 tablespoons chamomile leaves

Directions:

Make sure all the herbs you are using are dried and clean. Crush them into smaller pieces and set aside.

Line a tea ball with a paper towel so the finer bits of the herbs do not seep out of the ball as the tea is being prepared. Mix the herbs with 1 tablespoon black tea, and transfer to the ball.

Steep in a mug of hot water for up to 10 minutes, and stir in 1 tablespoon of honey, if desired. Enjoy.

Repeat up to 3 times per day for as long as symptoms persist.

This can also be used as a salve and be applied to the patient's neck and chest area. Repeat as often as needed for as long as symptoms persist.

Home Grown Health

What you will need:

1 tablespoon crushed dried burdock

1 tablespoon crushed ginger

Directions:

Make sure all the herbs you are using are dried and clean. Crush them into smaller pieces and set aside.

Line a tea ball with a paper towel so the finer bits of the herbs do not seep out of the ball as the tea is being prepared. Mix the herbs with 1 tablespoon black tea, and transfer to the ball.

Steep in a mug of hot water for up to 10 minutes, and stir in 1 tablespoon of honey, if desired. Enjoy.

Repeat up to 3 times per day for as long as symptoms persist.

Family's Choice

What you will need:

1 tablespoon marshmallow leaves

1 tablespoon licorice leaves

Directions:

Make sure all the herbs you are using are dried and clean. Crush them into smaller pieces and set aside.

Line a tea ball with a paper towel so the finer bits of the herbs do not seep out of the ball as the tea is being prepared. Mix the herbs with 1 tablespoon black tea, and transfer to the ball.

Steep in a mug of hot water for up to 10 minutes, and stir in 1 tablespoon of honey, if desired. Enjoy.

Repeat up to 3 times per day for as long as symptoms persist.

Aches Be Gone

What you will need:

1 tablespoon spearmint leaves

2 tablespoons crushed dried cilantro

8 drops tea tree oil

1/3 cup chopped beeswax

½ cup mango butter

Directions:

Heat 1 cup of water in a stainless steel pan on your stove. Crush the herbs and place them in the boiling water and turn the heat down to a simmer. Allow to simmer for 8 hours.

Strain the herbs out of the water and discard the herbs.

In a double boiler, melt the mango butter and beeswax. Once melted, stir in ½ cup of the herbal infused water. Add the tea tree oil next.

Once all is combined, transfer to another jar to cool.

Apply directly to infected area, and cover with a bandage. Wash the infected area with gentle soap and water and replace with more salve and a clean bandage twice per day.

Going Green
What you will need:

2 tablespoons clean, dried dandelion leaves

1 tablespoon crushed cumin seeds

Directions:

Make sure all the herbs you are using are dried and clean. Crush them into smaller pieces and set aside.

Line a tea ball with a paper towel so the finer bits of the herbs do not seep out of the ball as the tea is being prepared. Mix the herbs with 1 tablespoon black tea, and transfer to the ball.

Steep in a mug of hot water for up to 10 minutes, and stir in 1 tablespoon of honey, if desired. Enjoy.

Repeat up to 3 times per day for as long as symptoms persist.

It's a Health Thing
What you will need:

1 tablespoon dried fennel

2 tablespoons crushed valerian root

Directions:

Make sure all the herbs you are using are dried and clean. Crush them into smaller pieces and set aside.

Line a tea ball with a paper towel so the finer bits of the herbs do not seep out of the ball as the tea is being prepared. Mix the herbs with 1 tablespoon black tea, and transfer to the ball.

Steep in a mug of hot water for up to 10 minutes, and stir in 1 tablespoon of honey, if desired. Enjoy.

Repeat up to 3 times per day for as long as symptoms persist.

Wonder Tea

What you will need:

2 tablespoons dried ginseng

1 tablespoon dried orange zest

Directions:

Make sure all the herbs you are using are dried and clean. Crush them into smaller pieces and set aside.

Line a tea ball with a paper towel so the finer bits of the herbs do not seep out of the ball as the tea is being prepared. Mix the herbs with 1 tablespoon black tea, and transfer to the ball.

Steep in a mug of hot water for up to 10 minutes, and stir in 1 tablespoon of honey, if desired. Enjoy.

Repeat up to 3 times per day for as long as symptoms persist.

Salve Savior

What you will need:

1 tablespoon lavender

1 tablespoon holy basil

8 drops tea tree oil

1/3 cup chopped beeswax

½ cup mango butter

Directions:

Heat 1 cup of water in a stainless steel pan on your stove. Crush the herbs and place them in the boiling water and turn the heat down to a simmer. Allow to simmer for 8 hours.

Strain the herbs out of the water and discard the herbs.

In a double boiler, melt the mango butter and beeswax. Once melted, stir in ½ cup of the herbal infused water. Add the tea tree oil next.

Once all is combined, transfer to another jar to cool.

Apply directly to infected area, and cover with a bandage. Wash the infected area with gentle soap and water and replace with more salve and a clean bandage twice per day.

Better than Medicine
What you will need:

2 tablespoons dried mint leaves

1 tablespoon milk thistle

Directions:

Make sure all the herbs you are using are dried and clean. Crush them into smaller pieces and set aside.

Line a tea ball with a paper towel so the finer bits of the herbs do not seep out of the ball as the tea is being prepared. Mix the herbs with 1 tablespoon black tea, and transfer to the ball.

Steep in a mug of hot water for up to 10 minutes, and stir in 1 tablespoon of honey, if desired. Enjoy.

Repeat up to 3 times per day for as long as symptoms persist.

Sweet Dreams
What you will need:

2 tablespoons lavender leaves

1 tablespoon chamomile leaves

Directions:

Make sure all the herbs you are using are dried and clean. Crush them into smaller pieces and set aside.

Line a tea ball with a paper towel so the finer bits of the herbs do not seep out of the ball as the tea is being prepared. Mix the herbs with 1 tablespoon black tea, and transfer to the ball.

Steep in a mug of hot water for up to 10 minutes, and stir in 1 tablespoon of honey, if desired. Enjoy.

Repeat up to 3 times per day for as long as symptoms persist.

This can also be used as a salve and be applied to the patient's neck and chest area. Repeat as often as needed for as long as symptoms persist.

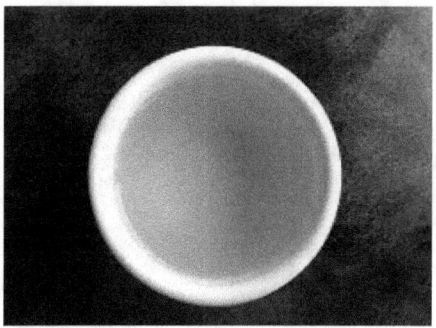

That's the Spot
What you will need:

2 tablespoons oregano

1 tablespoon dried parsley

8 drops tea tree oil

1/3 cup chopped beeswax

½ cup mango butter

Directions:

Heat 1 cup of water in a stainless steel pan on your stove. Crush the herbs and place them in the boiling water and turn the heat down to a simmer. Allow to simmer for 8 hours.

Strain the herbs out of the water and discard the herbs.

In a double boiler, melt the mango butter and beeswax. Once melted, stir in ½ cup of the herbal infused water. Add the tea tree oil next.

Once all is combined, transfer to another jar to cool.

Apply directly to infected area, and cover with a bandage. Wash the infected area with gentle soap and water and replace with more salve and a clean bandage twice per day.

School Days

What you will need:

1 tablespoon lemon mint leaves

1 tablespoon dried lemon zest

Directions:

Make sure all the herbs you are using are dried and clean. Crush them into smaller pieces and set aside.

Line a tea ball with a paper towel so the finer bits of the herbs do not seep out of the ball as the tea is being prepared. Mix the herbs with 1 tablespoon black tea, and transfer to the ball.

Steep in a mug of hot water for up to 10 minutes, and stir in 1 tablespoon of honey, if desired. Enjoy.

Repeat up to 3 times per day for as long as symptoms persist.

24 Hours Later

What you will need:

5 saffron florets

1 tablespoon passionflower leaves

Directions:

Make sure all the herbs you are using are dried and clean. Crush them into smaller pieces and set aside.

Line a tea ball with a paper towel so the finer bits of the herbs do not seep out of the ball as the tea is being prepared. Mix the herbs with 1 tablespoon black tea, and transfer to the ball.

Steep in a mug of hot water for up to 10 minutes, and stir in 1 tablespoon of honey, if desired. Enjoy.

Repeat up to 3 times per day for as long as symptoms persist.

Cool and Clear

What you will need:

1 tablespoon dried mint leaves

1 tablespoon dried peppermint leaves

8 drops tea tree oil

1/3 cup chopped beeswax

½ cup mango butter

Directions:

Heat 1 cup of water in a stainless steel pan on your stove. Crush the herbs and place them in the boiling water and turn the heat down to a simmer. Allow to simmer for 8 hours.

Strain the herbs out of the water and discard the herbs.

In a double boiler, melt the mango butter and beeswax. Once melted, stir in ½ cup of the herbal infused water. Add the tea tree oil next.

Once all is combined, transfer to another jar to cool.

Apply directly to infected area, and cover with a bandage. Wash the infected area with gentle soap and water and replace with more salve and a clean bandage twice per day.

Beautiful

What you will need:

1 tablespoon dried thyme

1 tablespoon dried rosemary

Directions:

Make sure all the herbs you are using are dried and clean. Crush them into smaller pieces and set aside.

Line a tea ball with a paper towel so the finer bits of the herbs do not seep out of the ball as the tea is being prepared. Mix the herbs with 1 tablespoon black tea, and transfer to the ball.

Steep in a mug of hot water for up to 10 minutes, and stir in 1 tablespoon of honey, if desired. Enjoy.

Repeat up to 3 times per day for as long as symptoms persist.

Back on Track

What you will need:

1 tablespoon turmeric

1 tablespoon cloves

Directions:

Make sure all the herbs you are using are dried and clean. Crush them into smaller pieces and set aside.

Line a tea ball with a paper towel so the finer bits of the herbs do not seep out of the ball as the tea is being prepared. Mix the herbs with 1 tablespoon black tea, and transfer to the ball.

Steep in a mug of hot water for up to 10 minutes, and stir in 1 tablespoon of honey, if desired. Enjoy.

Repeat up to 3 times per day for as long as symptoms persist.

No Place Like Health

What you will need:

1 tablespoon dried rose hips

2 tablespoons rosemary

8 drops tea tree oil

1/3 cup chopped beeswax

½ cup mango butter

Directions:

Heat 1 cup of water in a stainless steel pan on your stove. Crush the herbs and place them in the boiling water and turn the heat down to a simmer. Allow to simmer for 8 hours.

Strain the herbs out of the water and discard the herbs.

In a double boiler, melt the mango butter and beeswax. Once melted, stir in ½ cup of the herbal infused water. Add the tea tree oil next.

Once all is combined, transfer to another jar to cool.

Apply directly to infected area, and cover with a bandage. Wash the infected area with gentle soap and water and replace with more salve and a clean bandage twice per day.

Green Machine

What you will need:

2 tablespoons mint leave

1 teaspoon crushed coriander

Directions:

Make sure all the herbs you are using are dried and clean. Crush them into smaller pieces and set aside.

Line a tea ball with a paper towel so the finer bits of the herbs do not seep out of the ball as the tea is being prepared. Mix the herbs with 1 tablespoon black tea, and transfer to the ball.

Steep in a mug of hot water for up to 10 minutes, and stir in 1 tablespoon of honey, if desired. Enjoy.

Repeat up to 3 times per day for as long as symptoms persist.

Herbal Gurgle
What you will need:

1 tablespoon peppermint leaves

3 tablespoons chamomile leaves

Directions:

Make sure all the herbs you are using are dried and clean. Crush them into smaller pieces and set aside.

Line a tea ball with a paper towel so the finer bits of the herbs do not seep out of the ball as the tea is being prepared. Mix the herbs with 1 tablespoon black tea, and transfer to the ball.

Steep in a mug of hot water for up to 10 minutes, and stir in 1 tablespoon of honey, if desired. Enjoy.

Repeat up to 3 times per day for as long as symptoms persist.

Mother Nature's Favorite Healer

What you will need:

2 teaspoons turmeric

1 teaspoon black pepper

8 drops tea tree oil

1/3 cup chopped beeswax

½ cup mango butter

Directions:

Heat 1 cup of water in a stainless steel pan on your stove. Crush the herbs and place them in the boiling water and turn the heat down to a simmer. Allow to simmer for 8 hours.

Strain the herbs out of the water and discard the herbs.

In a double boiler, melt the mango butter and beeswax. Once melted, stir in ½ cup of the herbal infused water. Add the tea tree oil next.

Once all is combined, transfer to another jar to cool.

Apply directly to infected area, and cover with a bandage. Wash the infected area with gentle soap and water and replace with more salve and a clean bandage twice per day.

It's Scarcely a Scratch

What you will need:

1 tablespoon crushed cinnamon

1 tablespoon crushed garlic

8 drops tea tree oil

1/3 cup chopped beeswax

½ cup mango butter

Directions:

Heat 1 cup of water in a stainless steel pan on your stove. Crush the herbs and place them in the boiling water and turn the heat down to a simmer. Allow to simmer for 8 hours.

Strain the herbs out of the water and discard the herbs.

In a double boiler, melt the mango butter and beeswax. Once melted, stir in ½ cup of the herbal infused water. Add the tea tree oil next.

Once all is combined, transfer to another jar to cool.

Apply directly to infected area, and cover with a bandage. Wash the infected area with gentle soap and water and replace with more salve and a clean bandage twice per day.

When All Else Fails

What you will need:

2 teaspoons ground mustard

1 teaspoon black pepper

Directions:

Make sure all the herbs you are using are dried and clean. Crush them into smaller pieces and set aside.

Line a tea ball with a paper towel so the finer bits of the herbs do not seep out of the ball as the tea is being prepared. Mix the herbs with 1 tablespoon black tea, and transfer to the ball.

Steep in a mug of hot water for up to 10 minutes, and stir in 1 tablespoon of honey, if desired. Enjoy.

Repeat up to 3 times per day for as long as symptoms persist.

Doctor Green

What you will need:

1 teaspoon dried holy basil

1 tablespoon dried thyme

1 teaspoon rosemary leaves

Directions:

Make sure all the herbs you are using are dried and clean. Crush them into smaller pieces and set aside.

Line a tea ball with a paper towel so the finer bits of the herbs do not seep out of the ball as the tea is being prepared. Mix the herbs with 1 tablespoon black tea, and transfer to the ball.

Steep in a mug of hot water for up to 10 minutes, and stir in 1 tablespoon of honey, if desired. Enjoy.

Repeat up to 3 times per day for as long as symptoms persist.

Conclusion

There you have it, everything you need to know to make a variety of your own healing salves and teas – just by using all natural herbs. I hope this book was able to give you the inspiration you need to enjoy natural living, and that you mix up each and every one of these blends for your health today.

You can't put a price on your health, and you certainly don't want to fill your body with all those harmful side effects that you can experience from synthetic medicine. But now, you don't have to.

All these recipes are perfectly safe to use as much as you need to, giving you the power to control your health and enjoy your life while you save money, avoid chemicals, and much, much more.

I hope you feel inspired to change your life with this book, and that it gives you all the rich benefits you have been hoping for.

Happy healing.

FREE Bonus Reminder

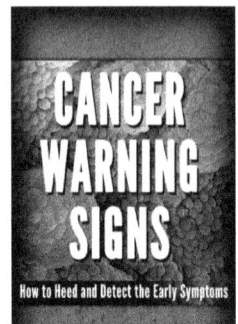

If you have not grabbed it yet, please go ahead and download your special bonus report *"DIY Projects. 13 Useful & Easy To Make DIY Projects To Save Money & Improve Your Home!"*

Simply Click the Button Below

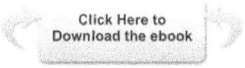

OR **Go to This Page**

http://healthylivingpeople.com/free/

BONUS #2: More Free & Discounted Books

Do you want to receive more Free & Discounted Books?

We have a mailing list where we send out our new Books when they go free or with a discount on Kindle. Click on the link below to sign up for Free & Discount Book Promotions.

=> Sign Up for Free & Discount Book Promotions <=

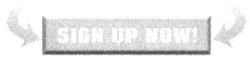

OR Go to this URL

http://zbit.ly/1WBb1Ek

www.ingramcontent.com/pod-product-compliance
Lightning Source LLC
Chambersburg PA
CBHW071309280526
45788CB00004B/1864